LOW CARB

DIET

TURNS FAT INTO ENERGY WITH PROTEIN DIET

ESSENTIAL BEGINNER'S GUIDE TO LOSE WEIGHT FAST

BALANCED FOOD PLAN AND RECIPES INCLUDED.

Claudia Rodriguez

Summary

INTRODUCTION

I looked at myself in the mirror, I was not satisfied with my body. I thought I deserved better, that body didn't represent me. Those little extra rolls made me feel very uncomfortable. For these reasons I started to go on different dieting paths. I needed to lose a few pounds, to accept myself more, to be satisfied with my body.

The first time I embarked on a diet was not easy at all. I have always had a very good relationship with food, in the sense that I have always loved to eat tasty food. With the first diet I embarked on, I realized that I could no longer eat many of the foods I loved. These severe restrictions led me to give up after a short time and fall back into my old bad habits.

I was not yet psychologically ready to seriously undertake a diet. This situation generated a feeling of frustration in me; I did not feel able to complete a goal I had set for myself. Usually in the other areas of my life I had always managed to achieve any goal but in this one the challenge had become very daunting.

Whenever I saw a cake or someone eating junk food in front of my eyes I could not resist, I knew it was wrong but staying away was very difficult.

For these reasons I used to try to eat healthily but as soon as I tasted those damned dishes again I would take 100 steps back, in fact I couldn't help myself, from one taste I would end up swallowing the whole plate.

Food had become a real drug for me. Fortunately I was and am a woman who moves a lot during the day, I would have risked being severely overweight. The real problem was that I could not detach myself. I started trying different diets in the hope of finding one that would make me miss food less, but each time I found myself back to square one.

By then I had almost given up hope when I first tried the Low Carb protein diet. This diet drastically changed my life for several reasons. Not only did it allow me to lose many kilograms in a very short time but also, and more importantly, to not suffer those very annoying and unmanageable feelings of lack of food. I did not feel hungry and in fact I did not even miss tasting the far from healthy food that was slowly destroying my body.

In this book I talk about this type of diet that drastically changed my life. Not only did I see myself in better shape after a short time but this also resulted in an increase in my self-confidence and allowed me to achieve better relationships with others.

The relationship with my home mirror has profoundly changed. If before it was my bitterest enemy after this diet it has become a friend. I have also learned to appreciate all my imperfections. My relationship with food has been completely transformed.

It is precisely for these reasons that I have decided to share with you in this handbook practical tips, weekly menus and quick recipes that can enable you to start on this path and achieve results that until recently you thought were unattainable.

Reading these pages will help you understand the diet you should really follow, what the pros are and how this differs from any other type of diet. I don't speak to you as a theoretician who has only and exclusively studied notions but everything I tell you I have tested on myself.

I must tell you, however, that before you take the first step on this new path you need to become aware of yourself, how important it is for you to lose weight and what it could mean for you.

The secret of everything do you know what it is? It is action.

Only by taking action can you change your destiny. So I ask you after reading this book not to stop at theory and apply all the notions that are written in these pages. You will enjoy trying different recipes and start following the menus that are given.

I can assure you that in just a few weeks you can see extraordinary results.

I ask you not to store this book in your bookshelf, do not let it gather dust. Despite its small size its value is very high, all the secrets of this diet are collected. I would like you to use it whenever you feel the need. Use it, underline what you think is important, crumple it, do what you want with it but don't leave it to its own devices. Prepare the recipes and follow step by step what I tell you.

We just have to delve into this new path.

Chapter 1 - LOVE YOURSELF AND FOOD.

Before starting any path it is important to love your body. Even if right now you cannot see yourself in the mirror or you are not satisfied with your physique, you should not be ashamed of it. Starting from this premise is very important. I read a story once that really struck me.

A professor came into the classroom with a €500 bill, took it in his hand and crumpled it, almost destroying it. Everyone looked at him puzzled, later exclaiming, "Who wants it?"

Everyone raised their hands despite the condition of the bill. Later the professor took it and pounded it under his feet and asked the same question again. This time, too, everyone raised their hand.

The moral of this story is that like the banknote at one point in your life you may believe that you are worthless, that you are not beautiful enough, that you are inferior to others but your value remains the same, like that of the banknote.

That is why even if you are not satisfied with your physique right now, you cannot repudiate it, you cannot hate it, you have countless reasons to love it instead.

However, it is also crucial to improve your relationship with food. Food is like gasoline for a car, without it it cannot run. Imagine now putting diesel into a gasoline car, what results would you get? You would destroy the engine. The moment you take the wrong food for your body all you do is damage it, without realizing it you are putting diesel rather than gasoline! In this book you will also learn how to follow a diet that can enable you to feed yourself properly and finally love your body.

Start loving your body because it is the only thing you have from the time you are born until you die. Be grateful to your body because it gives you the ability to move every day and always experience new sensations and emotions. The body that you so hate on some days is the same body that allows you to go to your friends to have fun, that allows you to achieve pleasure and also to do those little everyday things that might seem trivial. You cannot hate your body or yourself. When something breaks in your car what do you do? Do you repair it or throw the machine away? Don't think that destroying your body is the best solution. If it doesn't satisfy you, you must try to figure out how to improve your physical condition, but your love must remain unconditional. Also because we are all destined to grow old, to lose our muscles, to get our first stretch marks and wrinkles, this is nature but certainly that is not why we should hate our bodies.

Everyone has at least one reason to love their body; find yours. If you decide to hate your body all you are doing is wasting your energy in the wrong way. If you find yourself in this situation, which I also went through for a short time, I advise you to try to behave differently. As long as you do the same actions you will achieve the same results, so you have to act differently.

The real problem is that when a person is not satisfied with his or her body he or she also limits his or her mind. How many times have you avoided doing something with the desire to do it only at the time when you would lose weight. These conditions you set for yourself are completely wrong because all they do is limit your every action. Starting a diet that makes you lose weight and live fit is most important, but on the other hand you cannot limit your mind before you achieve any kind of result. For example, if you think with your mind that you should not go to the beach because you do not have a suitable physique or you should not put on a bikini, chase away these thoughts that only limit you and generate unhappiness and depression in you.

When negative feelings pervade our bodies we make it much more difficult to manage our nutrition and gorge ourselves on all kinds of foods that we should avoid. Basically, those who do not have a healthy diet in most cases are unhappy or dissatisfied with one aspect of their lives. That is why it becomes necessary before starting any kind of diet to start loving one's body, being well with oneself especially mentally. When this mental condition is achieved, unthinkable results can be achieved.

The mind is really the factor that drives people who are severely overweight to start exercising at some point in their lives and lose pounds. The mind has incredible power, so you have to make the most of it. Whenever you have a negative thought about yourself, chase it away, you deserve much better than these depowering thoughts.

From your birth as you know you live in your body, you can over time change its shape, be more fit at some times or overweight at others, you are the keeper of your body. Do you know what happens to a lot of people? When you receive a gift you are happy because it's something new, that you don't know about, but the moment the habit of having it overcomes you forget how great this is, the same happens with the body. People forget the potential of their body and not only neglect it but actually do everything to worsen its condition.

Actually your body you have had it and will have it for a long time but unlike gifts you cannot afford not to appreciate it. The more you devote your attention to it the more you will fall in love with it. Understanding what to eat, how to feed yourself properly, what diet to follow, really makes a difference in your life, which is why in this book I will tell you about the Low Carb Protein Diet. From the moment I gave up carbs and started eating healthy, I have loved myself a lot more and discovered that I have energy I didn't even imagine. Before I felt like a flooded car today instead I live in the body of a Ferrari.

After all, how could you not love your body, which is such a complex system that performs countless functions in every second: it pumps blood, allows your heart to beat, makes your eyelids flutter, regulates your body temperature, and more.

So before we delve into the most beloved diet ever start **loving yourself** too. Live in the moment, don't be a constant "work in progress," don't wait to change physically before you take action, start appreciating your life, only in this way will positive energy be released in you that will make it easier for you to follow this diet and achieve amazing results.

Chapter 2 - THE LOW CARB DIET, THE MOST LOVED DIET IN ABSOLUTE.

I don't deny it slimming down in a short time has always been my great desire, which I tried to make come true whenever I realized that I had gone a little overboard and had eaten out of control. I saw myself as out of shape and that was precisely why I wanted to find a remedy, obviously in the shortest possible time. This happened every time some occasion came at my door where it was important for me to be in shape, such as the upcoming summer or some ceremony or even just to see myself more beautiful in the mirror.

It was really embarrassing for me to show up in a bikini at the beach in front of other people, actually I had nothing to hide, I was simply a little out of shape however I couldn't see myself, so I strongly believed that everyone else made comments about my fitness.

Actually, let me let you in on a secret, most people do not have much time to spend in commenting on your physique. Maybe the moment they see something strange they talk about it for a few minutes, but soon after their minds are crowded with their own thoughts, which then cause them to turn their focus away from what they had previously seen.

This continuous feeling of discomfort has led me over the years to try so many diets on my own skin, on my own or even with the help of the best nutritionists, this has allowed me to become passionate about the subject and study day by day to learn a few more notions.

Today I can consider myself an expert in this area. In fact, I have had a lot of practice over time, almost as if before losing weight I really wanted to try them all.

I have to say that the diet that has given me the most results ever is the LOW CARB i.e., low-carbohydrate diet, also known as the protein diet.

Why is the LOW CARB diet so beloved?

Because it makes it possible to lose weight quickly and easily-that is, without the need to weigh food-by simply replacing carbohydrates and fats with protein.

This makes it easy for everyday life in that we can forget about obnoxious scales, calculating calories or weighing foods as in almost any other dietary regimen. Therefore, you will not have to be a little chemist, watching every little bit of food, but you will simply have to change your approach to it.

With this diet you will not suffer from hunger because you can also eat large amounts of food and at the same time achieve success in a short time. Yes, I know it sounds strange, it is not easy to believe something like this because most diets are based on microscopic amounts of food that should be ingested and give a sense of satiety.

What happens instead, in most cases, is that patients follow these diets with good results for a short period of time and then collapse psychologically and return to eating much larger amounts of food than before.

However, do not believe, given the great topicality of this diet, that it was born in recent decades; on the contrary, it boasts successes as early as the second half of the nineteenth century in the United States.

American doctors, in fact, had discovered the necessity of zeroing out carbohydrates in the daily diet to see rapid and lasting weight loss, a marked decrease in hunger and an improvement in the overall health of those who practiced it.

In fact, with regard to the latter aspect of health, we know how harmful an excess of sugars is to our bodies that can lead to diabetes, overweight and obesity in the long run. Obviously, low-carb diets go a long way toward eliminating refined sugars largely if not almost entirely from our diet, and the resulting benefits to our health are enormous. Imagine not only getting into great physical shape but also drastically improving your health, that would be nice wouldn't it? Well, the reality is that with this diet it is possible.

The protein diet also goes to almost completely eliminate two other substances, which are wheat and refined flours, and finally also fats. Undoubtedly this benefits our health.

It is in fact in baked goods, cakes, cookies, muffins, crackers, fast food such as chips, sandwiches and fried foods that the main sources of fat are contained. With the low carb diet, we are going to totally exclude these types of foods, this will result in a marked improvement in our health status.

It is clear that in order to achieve real results we must also avoid the consumption of alcohol and spirits, going to replace them in the case of cocktails or aperitifs with natural fruit juices, that is, extracts of fresh, seasonal fruits and vegetables that, in addition to avoiding the swelling typical of alcohol due to its vasoconstrictor effect, will also introduce fiber, vitamins and minerals into the body, which will also promote a beneficial antioxidant and purifying effect of accumulated toxins.

At the end of the day, does it really cost you that much to give up a cocktail with friends and have a juice or a centrifuged juice or even just a healthy sugar-free lemonade?

If you think about it I'm sure the answer will be "no, it's not that hard," so why don't you do it then? Start thinking in a healthy way for your body, don't conform to the masses simply to be conformist. Who knows that some of your friends seeing your choice will not copy you.

It is also best to avoid carbonated beverages and beer, the latter of which at most can be allowed in the alcohol-free version, as they contain gas and it is always better to prefer drinks that are free of it.

So eliminate all those drinks that are very common in fast food restaurants. For many this may be difficult but remember, the sooner you get used to it the sooner you will achieve the desired results.

During the diet, it is also necessary to drink a lot of water, again preferably natural and gas-free, which will therefore allow us to maintain proper hydration, going to decrease water retention and allowing us to purify ourselves both internally and externally and also going to promote satiety. You should not drink less than 2 liters of water a day, this is really the minimum amount. To have good hydration you should drink about 3 liters of water a day. Just think that for a period of my life I was drinking only 1 small bottle of water a day and maybe not even all of it actually....

Now since I have been constantly hydrating my life has completely changed, I can be more clear-headed and focus in both my work and personal life. If you are at work and carrying water mugs or large bottles can be difficult, I recommend you buy an aluminum water bottle, which are used a lot these days, and they also have a thermos function that allows you to keep the water temperature at the same level for a long time. So if you put fresh water in the water bottle, only after several hours will it become room temperature.

We are also allowed almost without limit in addition to water the use of herbal teas or natural infusions. I particularly recommend to combine with your diet the African red tea better known as Rooibos or white tea, both beverages are known not only for their very high antioxidant function but also for their slimming properties that is fat burning, and able to accelerate the metabolism that characterize them.

Green tea or draining or purifying herbal teas made from natural herbs are also excellent, the important thing is to drink them without added sugar, as they are already delicious as is, or at most you can add a sweetener such as Stevia or honey.

I must say that I myself consume Roobois red tea in my daily routine, I use the one in sachets which I find to be much more practical than the dried leaf tea. It can be purchased at any herbal or organic store. To enjoy this bagged tea, I steep it in a large pitcher so that it can last for several days and then sip it throughout the day. I myself have found its actual beneficial properties. I can assure you that the taste of Roobois red tea is not only unmistakable but excellent.

Therefore, we can argue that the numerous elements listed, such as assured and lasting weight loss and lack of hunger pangs, should make us love the protein diet, but in addition to that, this type of diet also allows us to activate our metabolism more, allowing us to burn calories and body fat faster and also going to increase our muscle mass.

In addition to this, the thing that made me personally love this type of diet so much was also the fact that the constant sense of hunger that gripped me all day long during other diets with this one totally disappeared; in fact, proteins have greater satiating power despite containing fewer calories.

As I also anticipated, because our bodies process protein foods more slowly, our metabolism stays more active and for longer thereby burning more calories and allowing us to lose more weight.

As for what kind of protein to take, having been a vegetarian myself for a period of time, for those who are, they will be able to safely substitute animal protein for plant protein. Being a vegetarian does not constitute any limitation to the protein diet, we will then see in more detail what foods to choose.

This is a diet suitable for everyone, any person regardless of age group, gender or lifestyle food choices.

☐

Chapter 3 - WHAT LOW CARB MEANS.

How can carbohydrates affect our weight? What effects do they have on our bodies? Is it really possible to minimize them?

To find out how the low carb protein diet works best, it is necessary first to go over the various functions that carbohydrates have for our bodies, that is, their effects both positive and negative.

Many times in fact, we are not really aware of what we ingest, plus we only hear about carbohydrates without knowing how they actually interact with our body.

Carbohydrate can be regarded as the nutrient that has the greatest influence in terms of raising blood sugar levels. This then results in increased insulin production by the body. This is a direct consequence. It therefore becomes essential for both diabetic and non-diabetic people to lower their blood sugar levels. Lowering insulin can help prevent a disease such as type 2 diabetes from occurring over time.

Insulin also has another task, that of storing fat in the body. This means that the moment we can reduce insulin in the body, we can lose weight much faster.

For our health, therefore, following a diet with lower carbohydrate content brings benefits not only to our physique, but also and especially to our health.

The first one is that we will be able to lose weight much faster, and it is the one that concerns the outward appearance the most. However, there are other very important benefits, such as:

-A lower chance of high sugar levels occurring.

-Lower risk of severe hypoglycemia

-More energy
-More mental clarity
-Lower risk of developing long-term health complications
But what is actually meant by low carbohydrate? Doctrine still does not unanimously agree on this concept, however, most believe that low carb means less than 130 g per day.

Very low carbohydrates, on the other hand, are defined as less than 30 grams per day.

It is important that you choose a level of carbohydrates that makes you feel good. Sometimes diets that are too extreme, that are far removed from what your eating habits are, can lead you to a high level of frustration, which is certainly not good for your body, and your mind.

In this book I will give you advice that is based on my experience that you can decide whether to follow or not, however, I recommend that before embarking on any diet path, you should consult with your doctor who will be able to give you some very important guidance especially if you are taking particular medications.

Returning to the role of carbohydrates for our bodies, they have a great influence, because just as proteins and fats act, carbohydrates also provide energy, so they fuel our bodies.

When we ingest carbohydrates, they are broken down during our digestion process into glucose, so there is an automatic increase in sugar, greater or lesser, depending on the amount ingested.

Ingesting a lower amount of carbohydrates allows you to tell your body that you do not need to produce such a high level of insulin. When there is a lower amount of insulin circulating in the body, it can help you prevent weight gain and indeed reduce it.

The items that are highest in carbohydrates are grains, fruits, vegetables, nuts, seeds, and legumes. We also generally ingest refined carbohydrates when we consume those found in white bread, cakes, sugary drinks and beverages, candy, cookies.

When I first found out about this I was quite upset. Every day without thinking about it I ate carbohydrates in large quantities believing that they were good for me, or at least that they could not have any negative effects on my health. In fact, we often believe that since everyone eats carbohydrates it is okay to do so.

I hope this paragraph opened your eyes as it did mine.

We are therefore going to minimize these kinds of foods by replacing them in a pleasant and varied way. Don't worry, we will see together step by step how to do it.

Carbohydrates are the main source of energy in the human body. They provide more than half of the total energy requirements and should make up about 50 percent of the diet, but below we will see how to succeed in maintaining a healthy energy balance, even by reducing them by a lot compared to these figures. Sometimes nutritionists even recommend including protein, fat and carbohydrates in the menu in a ratio of 1: 1: 4.

In the gastrointestinal tract, carbohydrates from food are broken down into simple sugars, which enter the bloodstream. A healthy adult's blood constantly contains about 6 g of glucose. This amount is enough to provide the body with energy for 15 minutes.

To maintain blood glucose at a normal level, the hormones insulin and glucagon are produced in the pancreas, which regulate blood glucose concentration, performing 2 completely opposite functions:

- Insulin lowers the increased amount of glucose in the blood by converting it to fat or glycogen. The latter is stored in the liver and muscles.
- Glucagon increases low blood glucose levels by converting glycogen into it.

Carbohydrates are divided into simple (fast) and complex (slow). The difference between them lies in the degree of complexity of the structural form of the molecules and the speed of assimilation. Simple carbohydrates include monosaccharides and disaccharides (fructose and glucose). They are immediately absorbed into the bloodstream, which leads to increased levels of glucose and insulin, which should neutralize it. With frequent and abundant consumption of foods rich in simple sugars, the pancreas may not bear the load and stop responding to an excessive rise in blood glucose concentration. This condition causes the development of type 1 diabetes mellitus, and blocks weight loss.

Complex carbohydrates also include polysaccharides. These are slowly broken down into simple sugars and gradually enter the bloodstream, providing a long and gradual supply of energy to the body. By eating foods rich in slow carbohydrates, a person is satiated for a long time and feels better because there are no spikes in blood glucose. In addition, fiber and pectins are nutrients for beneficial intestinal microflora, in fact through them one can improve peristalsis, digestion and cleansing the body of toxins.

For convenience, the usefulness and harmfulness of carbohydrate-containing foods can be determined by the glycemic index, which indicates the product's ability to raise blood glucose levels. Index 0 is assigned to food that contains no carbohydrates at all. Based on this, all foods are divided into 3 groups:
- High GI: 70 to 100.
- Average GI: 40 to 70.
- Low GI: 0 to 40.

The Low Carb diet therefore means reducing the number of carbohydrates to be consumed daily, so that when our body needs energy to perform an action, it does not draw from them but replenishes itself from the stores of fat in it.

How fats are turned into energy

In the Low Carb diet in addition to the low number of carbohydrates, it is also important to keep the level of fat introduced into the body low. Fats play a key role in our body, in fact they are used by our body to be converted into energy.

Fat is therefore a source of energy. However, when it is in excess, it accumulates in the body in the form of subcutaneous fat on the belly, particularly related to male obesity, and on the thighs and buttocks, mainly concerning female obesity. Fats perform three functions in the body: to give energy, to regulate (being used to form steroid hormones), and to build (i.e., constitute cell membranes).

One gram of fat contains 9.3 kcal, which is more than twice as much as one gram of carbohydrates or protein, but it is difficult for the body to obtain that energy.

The oxidation of fats is a multi-step process and is too expensive: it requires a lot of time and oxygen.

The body uses fat only at rest, or when working at low intensity. When you eat fats, your body does not use them immediately to produce energy, even during a diet. The only exception is when you eat a large amount of fat at a time (about 80 grams), but even then the effect is rather slight. All dietary fat is stored in fat cells every day. But if you are on a diet, fat from the reserves is gradually taken out to provide the body with the missing energy. This is precisely how diets such as low carb diets work; given the reduction in carbohydrate intake, the body will in fact be forced to draw from previously stored sources of fat; this will reduce the fat in our bodies and make us look drier and fitter.

So if there is excess energy in the body, which could be caused precisely by excess carbohydrate intake, it is deposited around the internal organs, and under the skin in the form of fatty tissue.

The process of fat burning in the scientific literature is called lipolysis. Under normal conditions, the body is accustomed to obtaining energy from carbohydrates.

But when a situation arises where there are not enough carbohydrates, our body starts looking for reserve sources. The fats stored in our body are just the right reserve stores that it will use.

Fat is a priority source of energy; there is always a sufficient amount of it in the body. If the intensity of work increases, the body first increases fat processing to the highest possible level, and only then connects other energy systems. Fats are digested into fatty acids and glycerol, and in this form they are oxidized by the mitochondria of cells during work or deposited in adipose tissue.

However, we must say that fats are essential for normal organ function, as well as for healthy bones, skin, and hair. Lack of healthy fats can negatively affect blood lipids, increase levels of bad cholesterol, and cause excessive absorption of fatty acids.

Low-fat diets should be approached with caution, which is why you need to be aware and conscious of what you are doing. Many low-fat foods have little or no flavor, and manufacturers sometimes add a lot of sugar, salt, and additives, so I advise you in all cases to read the labeling on any product you decide to consume.

Fat, however, unlike what is often thought, cannot be burned simply by sweating, such as perhaps by spending time in a sauna. In fact, when you sweat in a sauna, all you are doing is consuming body fluids, but you are not going to burn fat, because you are not in a stressed condition. That is why it is necessary to understand how to consume fat.

During our daily routine, any movement we make requires energy costs. The main energy molecule is ATP (adenosine triphosphoric acid) from which calories are generated, this is formed by the breakdown of carbohydrates and fats.

During physical exertion, first of all, carbohydrates "burn" with the formation of energy ATP. These compounds are the simplest and most accessible, since they are constantly in the blood plasma.

With a decrease in their concentration, the body begins to use accumulated reserves. Simple blood sugar is sufficient for only 10 minutes of aerobic exercise.

With aerobic exercise, the most important thing is to control breathing, as the appearance of shortness of breath leads to a lack of oxygen, which is necessary for the process of burning calories.

Energy reserves include two main compounds: glycogen and fat. As for muscle fibers, the more developed they are in the body, the less time it takes to deplete muscle glycogen reserves. After the energy stored from the above sources is depleted, liver glycogen begins to be metabolized.

The second source of glucose when lowered in the blood is fat catabolism. This is much more complicated than the breakdown of glycogen, and takes longer. Because first fat, breaking down into triglycerides and fatty acids, is released into the bloodstream from lipids and only then, once it enters muscle cells, it burns up into kilocalories, being metabolized into glucose.

In the training process, fat metabolism begins only after about an hour of exercise. Then, after exercise, muscles restore glycogen deficiency at the expense of body fat. Static and power loads lead to an increase in muscle mass, which, in turn, increases energy expenditure and accelerates fat burning. The greater the muscle mass, the greater the energy required to work the muscles, so fat burning is greatly accelerated.

The most effective fat-burning exercise is cardio loading, since the constant dynamic work of the muscles requires more energy. This includes:

Jogging: during the first 20 minutes, glucose is burned, as measured jogging involves many muscles in our body, so fat catabolism is related to correcting ATP deficiency.

Deep and even breathing (no shortness of breath) allows the blood to be sufficiently oxygenated, improving energy metabolism. Practicing this also trains the cardiovascular system, which is activated for sufficient blood supply, and effective skeletal muscle work.

Dancing: dynamic and complex movements to the rhythm of music are effective. Also, during dancing, the amount of endorphins in the blood (the pleasure hormone) increases, which speeds up metabolic processes and reduces the feeling of fatigue, increasing efficiency.

Swimming: with the right technique, almost all muscles are involved in this sport. Because water is denser than air, and more force is needed to move the muscle, the caloric intake burned is increased. Unfortunately, not everyone has access to this method of fat burning, as sufficient lung volume and the skills of proper water breathing are required for sufficient oxygen supply, since calorie burning under anaerobic conditions is impossible.

Riding a bicycle: this is a good alternative to jogging because in addition to working the leg muscles, it also works the core muscles that are used to maintain balance.

Body building: there is no denying the effectiveness of strength training in the gym as well, although here to have a fat-burning effect, alternating short, intense training for muscle growth with more effective aerobic exercise, such as circuit training, is necessary to maximize fat loss, as aerobic training requires more energy and more fat is burned.

Chapter 4 - THE CHOICE OF FOODS: WHICH TO PREDICT.

Having established at this point that eating protein foods burns more calories, and there is an activation of our metabolism, and that protein having greater satiating power makes the famous hunger pangs that characterize all other diets disappear, let us now delve into what foods to introduce to best follow this type of diet.

The foods richest in protein are lean meat and fish, the latter of which we should prefer in our weekly menu to meat, as it is rich in Omega 3 i.e., fatty acids that are great for the health of our body and can be found on salmon, shrimp, sardines, mackerel, walnuts, flaxseed and vegetables and are perfect for protein diets. These are all types of fish that can be found very easily in any supermarket or market.

As for meat certainly our choice should be lean meat such as turkey or chicken and beef, because fatty meats should be carefully avoided for our menus as they can lead in the long run to cardiovascular disease or related disorders.

In addition to lean meat and fish we can eat eggs and green leafy vegetables, also low-fat dairy products and cheeses, such as low-fat but protein-rich cottage cheese, light mozzarella or low-fat Greek yogurt, preferably it is important in general that it is labeled with no added sugar.

Protein shakes or shakes can also be included in our diet but I recommend taking these only on special days when one does not have time to take a meal leisurely due to impending family or work commitments, but it should remain 'one-time' and not become a habit as although rich in nutrients and vitamins these types of meal replacements are not suitable for continued use and healthy eating.

In any case in case one decides to replace a meal with a protein shake one should prefer to consume it at dinner, this is because the next morning having not taken in any carbohydrates at all one will certainly find oneself feeling less hungry and the protein contained therein will also be more assimilated by our body as we sleep through the night.

I myself sometimes use protein shakes due to lack of time and the need for a quick meal, but again I recommend being careful which ones to choose, because there are also many poor quality protein powders on the market so when buying them make sure they contain high quality raw materials and also essential vitamins and minerals to ensure you get the right nutrients.

About the protein diet, it is a commonplace to think that in the long run practicing it can bring us kidney problems.

Nothing could be more wrong, in fact it is actually just a generalized belief and there are no scientific studies to prove it. It is clear that if someone suffers from kidney disease perhaps this diet is not very suitable, but if we instead keep our diet balanced and enrich it with Omega 3 and then also with dried fruits such as nuts or almonds and again with green leafy vegetables and low-sugar fruits, we will certainly succeed in creating a correct and healthy diet that will lead us to keep fit without creating any kind of health problems for ourselves.

So if you, like me and like almost all women and often men as well, have tried a plethora of diets you certainly are aware that in each one there are foods that are forbidden and in the case of this one for sure they are the carbohydrate-rich foods such as pasta, bread, rice and potatoes.

It is very easy to remember which foods to eliminate, almost as if it were a child's game, these in fact are all those that begin with the letter P: pasta, pizza, bread, piadina, potatoes etc.

Another type of foods that are allowed but need to be careful about are fatty cold cuts such as salami, sausage and bologna, which in fact certainly contain a lot of protein but are also foods that are high in salt and saturated fat and therefore promote water retention and cellulite and many other related disorders so you should definitely not overdo these.

Chapter 5 - PROTEIN FOODS YES AND NO.

What specifically are the foods allowed and those to be eliminated in our protein regimen at this point?

FOODS ALLOWED IN THE PROTEIN DIET:

- **FISH**: tuna, salmon, cod, sardines, mackerel, mussels, shellfish.

You can eat fish even 3 or 4 times a week, the cooking I recommend in the weekly menu is either in a nonstick pan so that the use of cooking fat is minimal, or grilled or baked or boiled.

For quantities, portions can range from 150 g to 200 g.

- **LEAN MEAT**: chicken, turkey, beef or veal.

You can consume it 2 or 3 times a week with recommended cooking as above or in a nonstick skillet or grilled or baked.

- **Lean meats**: defatted raw ham, defatted cooked ham, bresaola, turkey rump.

These can preferably be consumed no more than twice a week, in portions ranging from 80 to 100 g.

- **EGGS**: are very rich in protein, advisable to consume especially the yolks, can be included in the diet up to 4 times a week, cooking can be soft-cooked, hard-boiled or in the form of omelet.

- **Dairy products**: low-fat low-fat such as light dairy flakes, light mozzarella cheese, grana cheese, low-fat Greek yogurt, light fresh cheeses, cottage cheese preferably sheep's milk or otherwise light. The recommended serving size for milk, yogurt or fresh cheeses is about 150 ml or gr.
- **VEGETABLE MILK**: oat, almond, rice or soy **milk** preferably without added sugar, about 150 ml per serving.
- **VEGETABLE YOGURT**: any yogurt with vegetable milk the important thing here is to avoid products with added sugars as well.
- **GREEN LEAF VEGETABLES**: excellent for maintaining good health and a good eating lifestyle. They are the vegetables such as spinach, salad greens such as lettuce, arugula, envy and valerian, and again chard, celery, broccoli, cauliflower and savoy cabbage are vegetables in fact rich in potassium but low in sodium and rich in antioxidants that make them a panacea for our body.

For vegetarian people are also recommended...
- **FOODS RICH IN PROTEIN DERIVED FROM SOYBEANS** such as: burgers, vegetables, dehydrated soybeans, tofu, tempeh.
- **FOODS RICH IN PROTEIN DERIVED FROM FRUIT**: seitan, which can be found in so many preparations such as frankfurters, sliced or stew.

I also advise meat-eaters not to skip this type of plant-protein-rich foods outright, because as I mentioned earlier, since we cannot overburden our bodies with excessive consumption of meat, especially red meat, these types of foods are an excellent plant-based alternative and also allow us to create a richer varied and healthy diet.

Other foods that vegetarians can eat on this type of diet include, for example: seitan and edamame.

Regarding seitan, we immediately say that it should be avoided by people who suffer from celiac disease and are gluten intolerant.

It is a very popular source of protein for both vegans and vegetarians. It contains a lot of gluten, which is the main protein in wheat. In appearance and texture it closely resembles well-cooked meat.

Every 100 grams contains about 25 grams of protein, almost the same protein levels as meat, numbers that are nothing short of incredible when you consider that it does not come from an animal source. It also contains small amounts of iron, calcium and phosphorus. It is a highly recommended alternative to meat, both for vegetarians and also for people who want to vary their diet more but at the same time eat foods with good nutritional values.

Edamame, on the other hand, are immature soybeans. They have a sweet, slightly grassy flavor that is very distinctive, making their taste easily recognizable. In fact, they differ from all other foods that have a high protein value. Before eating them, it is advisable to steam or boil them. They should be eaten on their own or are also highly recommended with soups and salads to give them a very special and natural taste.

They contain high levels of iron, calcium and about 10 grams of protein per 100 grams. They have much lower values than the seitan I described above, however they are a very good food that can be best integrated into the diet.

FOODS ALLOWED AT REDUCED CONSUMPTION:

- **INTEGRAL PRODUCTS**: preferable among these is 100% whole grain rye bread.
- **DRIED FRUIT**: such as walnuts, pine nuts, peanuts, cashews, Brazil nuts and pistachios, to be included because they are rich in Omega 3 but to be consumed in small amounts because they are also rich in fat anyway.
- **OILSEEDS**: sunflower seeds, flax seeds, sesame seeds and pumpkin seeds, which are also rich in Omega 3 but should also be used in moderate amounts because they are also rich in fat.
- **LEGUMES**: such as lentils, chickpeas, beans, peas, broad beans, and edamame are high-protein plant foods, but since they also contain quite a few carbohydrates we include them in this group, recommended, without overdoing it, for those who are vegetarians; they can be eaten in various ways. They can be boiled au naturel with a drizzle of extra virgin olive oil or blended or even cooked in the form of soups or velvety soups or in the form of veggie burgers and patties.
- Fructose-reduced ORANGE **FRUIT**: such as lemons and oranges, which are rich in vitamin C, have a high antioxidant and anti-aging function and contribute to the formation of new collagen for the skin.
- **RED FRUITS**: such as raspberries, blackberries and blueberries. Among other things, the red fruits just listed are very rich in antioxidants so they are a panacea for the prevention of skin aging and for a healthy diet.

- **WHITE or GREEN FRUIT**: Like apple, kiwi and lime, these fruits are also recommended because they are rich in antioxidants and vitamins.

ARE INSTEAD TO BE CONSIDERED PROHIBITED

-**SWEETS**
-**FATTY MEATS**.
-**WHITE FLOUR PRODUCTS**: bread, pasta, pizza, piadina, sweet and savory pastry products, etc.
-**FOODS RICH IN CARBOHYDRATES**: rice, potatoes, carrots, corn, etc.
-**FATTY FOODS** : aged cheeses, cream, mascarpone, etc.
-**HIGH FRUIT FRUIT CONTENT**: figs, mangoes, grapes, cherries, etc.
So summing up what can we eat?
Many things can be eaten, certainly the best proteins to take are the lean meats of chicken and turkey without the skin, all types of fish indicated, beef preferably in lean cuts, low-fat dairy products, eggs especially egg whites, and for all people who prefer vegetable proteins tofu, seitan and all other soy-based meat substitutes. We can also eat all the vegetables indicated, and among fats, extra virgin olive oil, nuts in small amounts, and avocados are preferred.
Among the recommended fats, I want to pause and talk about a fat that I love very much, which is **COCONUT OIL**.
You may have heard of coconut oil as a "bad" fat for our cardiovascular health and harmful to the body.

Forget all that because not only is coconut oil a good and healthy fat, but it can also become an ally in our diet, and it is also one of my dietary secrets in addition to my daily consumption of Robois red tea. Every morning I ingest a couple of tablespoons of coconut oil on an empty stomach before breakfast.

You can find it in organic stores either in jar in solid form that should be stored in the refrigerator, or in bottle in oily form. I prefer the latter because in my opinion it is easier to administer but it is up to you to choose which you prefer as the benefits of both are absolutely identical.

Why then do I recommend introducing it into your routine and daily routine?

Because the medium-chain triglycerides better known as MCTs contained in coconut oil create a long-term energy release by also going to speed up our metabolism and promoting fat loss, it also releases its nutrients slowly providing us with a long-term energy reserve by decreasing hunger and helping us burn fat particularly in the waist area.

Chapter 6 - THE PROTEIN DIET WEEKLY MENU.

Let us now look at the weekly menu of the protein diet, which will allow us if we do not indulge in carbohydrates or sugars to lose weight in a short time without regaining weight.

Clearly, this menu can be repeated for 14 days or even longer, you just need to reverse the meals or combine them to your liking.

I also recommend that you always have all the meals indicated, including snacking and snacking, in fact this will ensure that by eating often your metabolism will always remain active and you will certainly arrive at the main meals less hungry, and this will also benefit your diet and weight loss.

So let's see together what meals you will need to eat day by day. For each time of day, I have provided you with several options so that you can choose which one you prefer according to your tastes.

Do not immediately follow a drastic diet that is completely different from your eating habits because it could generate a lot of stress in you from such a situation, and it could push you to eat again in a way that is deleterious to your body.

So I advise you to choose options really based on your preferences and initially not to be too rigid with yourself.

Day 1: Monday

Breakfast
Option 1: Tea or latte with semi-skimmed milk + one low-fat Greek white or fruit yogurt
Option 2: Coffee + scrambled eggs (one red and two white) with a tiny bit of tomato pulp added if desired.
Snack
Option 1: One orange juice or grapefruit or orange juice without sugar
Option 2: A fresh seasonal fruit preferably from among the recommended ones
Lunch
Option 1: fish of your choice of cod (fillets found frozen are also fine) or sea bass or sea bream or sole cooked in a nonstick pan with a drizzle of raw olive oil + side dish of your choice of boiled vegetables you can choose from spinach or chard or kale or cabbage or broccoli
Option 2: 150 g light cheese of your choice of mozzarella or ricotta light or primosale, and as a side dish two fennels in pinzimonio with a drizzle of oil and salt or mixed salad.
Snack: low-fat white or fruit yogurt
Dinner: grilled chicken breast + side dish of your choice of boiled vegetables you can choose from spinach or chard or kale or cabbage or broccoli or as a side dish fennel in a dip with oil and salt or even mixed salad.

Day 2: Tuesday

Breakfast
Option 1: Coffee or latte with semi-skimmed milk + one low-fat or white Greek yogurt or fruit yogurt
Option 2: Milk with whole grain oatmeal or muesli of your choice without sugar.
Snack
Option 1: fresh fruit
Option 2: Low-fat white or fruit yogurt.
Lunch
Option 1: Fat-free ham or fat-free cooked ham + a slice of 100% whole-wheat rye bread toasted + vegetable of your choice of grilled red radicchio or mixed salad
Option 2: 2 omelet eggs with grated parmesan cheese + spinach or grilled tomatoes or mushrooms or other vegetables of choice.
Snack: a fruit or low-fat yogurt.
Dinner: fish either pan-fried or baked in your choice of salmon or cod or sardines or sea bass or trout + grilled eggplant or zucchini on a nonstick skillet with a drizzle of olive oil and a slice of toasted whole-wheat rye bread.

Day 3: Wednesday

Breakfast
Option 1: Coffee or latte with semi-skimmed milk + one low-fat Greek white or fruit yogurt
Option 2: Scrambled eggs (one red and two white) + a juice or orange or grapefruit juice without sugar

Snack
Option 1: One fruit or low-fat yogurt
Option 2: A small handful of dried fruits.
Lunch
Option 1: Grilled chicken breast or turkey breast + vegetables of your choice of mixed salad or grilled peppers
Option 2: 150gr light cheese + boiled fennel or zucchini vegetables seasoned with a drizzle of olive oil and enough salt and pepper.
Snack
Option 1: One low-fat white or fruit yogurt
Option 2: A fresh seasonal fruit.
Dinner: minestrone or vegetable puree are also good ones that can be purchased from among the frozen foods listed as 'light' + a 30-gram piece of grana cheese + boiled vegetables of your choice of spinach or broccoli or cauliflower or fresh fennel in a dip.

Day 4: Thursday

Breakfast
Option 1: Coffee or latte with semi-skimmed milk + one low-fat Greek white or fruit yogurt
Option 2: yogurt + whole grain oatmeal or blueberries.
Snack
Option 1: Orange juice or a sugar-free fruit juice or orange or pineapple or grapefruit.
Option 2: A fresh fruit.
Lunch
Option 1: Sliced grilled beef or turkey breast or chicken with mixed salad or boiled vegetables with your choice of cauliflower or broccoli or cabbage or spinach.

Option 2: 2 hard-boiled eggs + tuna without oil + mixed salad or boiled vegetables of your choice of cauliflower or broccoli or spinach.
Snack
Option 1: A low-fat yogurt and a piece of granola.
Option 2: One fruit.
Dinner:
Option1: Smoked salmon carpaccio (you buy ready smoked salmon and put it on the plate) with songino (lamb's lettuce) salad on top and various seeds on top
Option 2: Vegetable puree + 30 g grain + green salad or boiled vegetables spinach or chard or cauliflower or broccoli.

Day 5: Friday

Breakfast
Option 1: Coffee or latte with semi-skimmed milk + one low-fat or white Greek yogurt or fruit yogurt.
Option 2: Whole grain oat muesli with blueberries or scrambled eggs +squeezed orange juice or a glass of sugar-free orange juice.
Snack
Option 1: one low-fat yogurt
Option 2: One fruit
Lunch:
Option 1: Bresaola with arugula and cherry tomatoes
 Option 2: sliced turkey rump with arugula and cherry tomatoes + a 100g slice of whole grain rye bread

Snack
Option 1: A low-fat yogurt or fruit

Option 2: A small handful of dried fruits.
Dinner
Option 1: Boiled or grilled fish of your choice of cod or sole or sea bass + grilled vegetables of your choice of eggplant radicchio or zucchini.
Option 2: A big salad of tuna without oil + hard-boiled egg + tomato and green salad.

Day 6: Saturday

Breakfast
Option 1: Coffee or coffee and milk with semi-skimmed milk + one low-fat or white Greek yogurt or fruit yogurt.
Option 2: Scrambled eggs + a glass of sugar-free orange or grapefruit juice or sugar-free muesli + low-fat white yogurt.
Snack
Option 1: One low-fat white or fruit yogurt.
Option 2: One fruit of your choice.
Lunch
Option 1: light mozzarella caprese + tomato + fresh fennel pinzimonio
Option 2: Grilled salmon or other fish plus boiled vegetables of your choice of spinach or cauliflower or chard or green salad.
Snacks
Option 1: A low-fat yogurt or fruit
Option 2: A small handful of dried fruits.
Dinner
Option 1: Egg omelet with asparagus or zucchini or tomatoes + grilled vegetables with your choice of zucchini or peppers or tomato or eggplant.

Option 2: Meat or fish carpaccio with arugula and parmesan shavings.

As previously mentioned these are menu directions that can be by you then combined as you like the important thing is to balance the consumption of meat and fish and the other nutrients. You may have noticed that the menus I have proposed are 6 days, because I have left one day a week as a **"cheat day**," that is, a day off so that you can 'splurge' without obviously overdoing it.

You can then eat whatever you most desire such as a pizza or a "free" appetizer without restrictions. In fact, it is a proven fact that providing for one day's pick-me-up per week will help those on a diet to then more enthusiastically resume the next day the weight loss goal they had set for themselves.

WEEKLY VEGETARIAN MENU

Below I also offer the menu for those who are vegetarian and want to follow the protein diet thus going to replace meat or fish with non-animal foods.

Day 1: Monday

Breakfast
Option 1: Tea or latte with part-skim milk or vegetable soy milk or almond milk or oat milk + one low-fat Greek white or fruit yogurt.

Option 2: Coffee + scrambled eggs (one red and two white) with a tiny bit of tomato pulp added if desired.

Snack

Option 1: One orange juice or grapefruit or orange juice without sugar.

Option 2: A fresh seasonal fruit preferably among the recommended ones.

Lunch

Option 1: Grilled seitan + side dish of your choice of boiled vegetables you can choose from spinach or chard or cabbage or broccoli.

Option 2: Grilled veggie burgers + pickled fennel with a drizzle of oil and salt or mixed salad.

Snack: one low-fat white or fruit yogurt

Dinner: 150gr light cheese of your choice + side dish of your choice from boiled vegetables, you can choose from spinach or chard or kale or cabbage or broccoli or as a side dish fennel in a dip with oil and salt or even mixed salad.

Day 2: Tuesday

Breakfast

Option1: Coffee or latte with semi-skimmed milk or vegetable milk of your choice + one low-fat or white Greek yogurt or fruit yogurt.

Option 2: Milk with whole grain oatmeal or muesli of your choice without sugar.

Snack

Option 1: A fresh fruit.

Option 2: One low-fat white or fruit yogurt.

Lunch: 70 g whole-wheat buckwheat or whole-wheat spelt pasta topped with pachino or datterino tomatoes sautéed in a pan with a drizzle of olive oil and basil + vegetables of your choice of grilled red radicchio or spinach or grilled tomatoes or mushrooms.

Snack: a fruit or low-fat yogurt.

Dinner: grilled tofu + grilled eggplant or zucchini on nonstick pan with a drizzle of olive oil and a 100 g slice of toasted whole-wheat rye bread.

Day 3: Wednesday

Breakfast

Option 1: Coffee or latte with semi-skimmed milk or vegetable milk of your choice + one low-fat Greek white or fruit yogurt.

Option 2: Scrambled eggs (one red and two white) + a juice or orange or grapefruit juice without sugar

Snack

Option 1: A seasonal fruit

Option 2: A low-fat yogurt or a small handful of dried fruit.

Lunch

Option 1: 70 g brown rice seasoned with a little oil + vegetables of your choice of mixed salad or grilled peppers or zucchini

Option 2: 2 omelet eggs with parmesan cheese + boiled fennel dressed with a drizzle of olive oil and salt and pepper or mixed salad.

Snacks

Option 1: One low-fat white or fruit yogurt.

Option 2: A fresh seasonal fruit.

Dinner: minestrone or vegetable puree are also good ones that can be purchased among the frozen foods listed as 'light'or other light soup of your choice + a 30-gram piece of granola + boiled vegetables of your choice of spinach or broccoli or cauliflower or fresh fennel.

Day 4: Thursday

Breakfast
Option 1: Coffee or latte with semi-skimmed milk or vegetable milk of your choice + one low-fat Greek white or fruit yogurt
Option 2: Whole grain oatmeal with blueberries.
Snack
Option 1: fresh squeezed orange juice or sugar-free fruit juice
Option 2: Fresh centrifuge or a fresh seasonal fruit.
Lunch: 70 g couscous or whole-wheat buckwheat pasta or whole-wheat spelt pasta topped with a drizzle of olive oil and vegetables of your choice + mixed salad or boiled vegetables or chard or kale or spinach.
Snack
Option 1: One low-fat white or fruit yogurt
Option 2: One fruit of your choice in season.
Dinner
Option 1: 1 light mozzarella cheese + hard-boiled eggs + salad or valerian or arugula and a sprinkling of flax or sesame or poppy seeds
Option 2: Vegetable puree + 30 g grain + green salad or boiled vegetables spinach or chard or cauliflower or broccoli or mixed salad.

Day 5: Friday

Breakfast
Option 1: Coffee or latte with part-skim milk +one low-fat Greek or white or fruit yogurt or whole grain oat muesli with blueberries.
Option 2: Scrambled eggs +orange juice or a glass of sugar-free orange juice.
Snack: a low-fat yogurt or fruit
Lunch:70g chickpeas or lentils with arugula and cherry tomatoes and parmesan + a 100g slice of whole grain rye bread
Snack
Option 1: A low-fat yogurt or fruit.
Option 2: A small handful of dried fruits.
Dinner
Option 1: 2 veggie burgers of your choice or grilled seitan + grilled vegetables of your choice of eggplant radicchio or zucchini.
Option 2: A big salad of light mozzarella cheese + hard-boiled eggs + tomatoes and green salad.

Day 6: Saturday

Breakfast
Option 1: Coffee or coffee and milk with semi-skimmed milk or vegetable milk of your choice + one low-fat or white Greek yogurt or fruit yogurt.

Option 2: Scrambled eggs + a glass of sugar-free orange or grapefruit juice or sugar-free muesli + low-fat white yogurt.

Snack

Option 1: low-fat white or fruit yogurt

Option 2: Fresh blueberries or a fresh fruit

Lunch:

Option 1: light mozzarella caprese+ tomatoes+ fresh fennel pinzimonio

Option 2: 70 g boiled chickpeas or beans plus grilled vegetables of your choice of zucchini or eggplant or tomatoes or green salad.

Snacks

Option 1: One low-fat yogurt.

Option 2: One fruit

Dinner:

Option 1: scrambled egg omelet with zucchini or tomatoes or asparagus + vegetables to taste

Option 2: 2 veggie burgers or grilled seitan or tofu + green salad or boiled vegetables.

Chapter 6 - VARIATING THE PROTEIN DIET WITH EASY AND QUICK RECIPES.

Do you ever try to go on a diet but realize only later that you don't have time to prepare all the dishes you should be eating?

I confess that I myself being very busy for work have found myself in this unpleasant situation many times.

Initially I tried to do everything to follow the diet meticulously however after a short time this became really stressful for me and without realizing it I would go back to eating junk food, resuming those bad habits from which I was trying to get away in every way.

I generally do not have much time to cook, despite that I like to take care of myself and vary often in the kitchen to avoid getting tired of eating the same things over and over again. Over time, I have managed to find quick and easy recipes to prepare, so called balanced eating without going crazy with calculations and calories, so that I can make a ready-made, dietary meal in just a few minutes.

After preparing these dishes in a short time, my eating regimen changed drastically (for the better).

Therefore, below are some recipes that are easy to make and with the possibility of varying the basic ingredients to make ever-changing menus. The quantities given are for one person but can be changed.

For example, if you cook for two or three people you can double or triple the amounts. I recommend that you never lack some basic ingredients for a healthy and light diet at home to avoid later resorting in times of need to the classic plate of pasta to appease hunger in a short time or the classic order on JustEat of junk food.

You will simply have to keep some chicken or turkey breast in the freezer, some lean beef burgers, some fresh vegetables in the refrigerator such as tomatoes or salad or frozen spinach, and in any eventuality we will be safe without endangering our diet.

As for the seasoning I recommend that you always use the HIMALAYA PINK salt as your seasoning, my recommendation is in fact to buy this type of salt in both "fine" and "coarse" versions and always substitute it for ordinary table salt.

In fact, Himalayan pink salt is not refined and is never treated with any process where chemicals are used, and it also remains by its nature free of the pollutants that can instead contaminate types of salt that come from seas and oceans.

It also seems to reduce water retention and hypertension because its sodium chloride content is significantly lower than ordinary table salt. So even though the cost is a little higher than ordinary salt, it is worth buying. After all, as the German philosopher Feuerbach said, "We are what we eat," so it is worth spending a little more to improve our diet and consequently our health.

As for the oil I recommend that you always use a good evo oil i.e. Extra Virgin Olive Oil, and hereafter I will always use the abbreviation evo oil to mean precisely extra virgin olive oil.

Here are some recipes that can come in very handy during your dieting period.

STRACCETTI WITH ARUGULA AND CHERRY TOMATOES

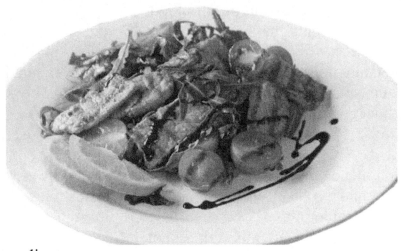

Ingredients:
-150 g slices of lean veal, also perfect for carpaccio, or chicken or turkey breast.
-100g pre-washed salad arugula or lamb's lettuce (songino)
-10 pachino or date tomatoes.
Take the chosen meat and cut it with kitchen scissors into thin strips. Afterwards cook it in a nonstick pan with a little water, once cooked add arugula or lamb's lettuce and put on the cherry tomatoes previously cut into coarse pieces, season with salt and enough evo oil.

GRILLED CHILI BEEF WITH AVOCADO

Ingredients:
-150 g lean rump of beef
-¼ clove of crushed garlic

-20 ml of red wine
-1 touch of dried chili flakes
-50 g avocado made into slices
-Half a basil leaf
-1/3 chopped cucumber
-Thin slices of onion
-1 teaspoon oil
-Half tablespoon of vinegar and red wine

To prepare this dish you will have to put in a bowl, all together: garlic, red wine and chili in the sizes I have indicated. You will have to mix everything and dip the steak in it and keep it in the refrigerator for 10 minutes, this you need to make the marinade.

While this bowl is in the refrigerator start making the avocado salad. To do this you will need to combine the avocado with the basil, cucumber and red onion in one bowl. Next add the olive oil and vinegar and mix everything together.

Now all you have to do is heat a lightly greased nonstick skillet over medium-high heat. When this is hot, after a few seconds, you should add the steak and cook it 5 minutes on each side. The result will be a steak that is slightly charred on the outside and cooked medium-rare on the inside. Now that you have cooked the steak you can garnish the dish with the avocado salad you prepared earlier.

SALMON OR TUNA CARPACCIO WITH VALERIAN AND CRISPY ALMONDS

Ingredients:
-100   g packaged smoked salmon or tuna,

-100   g valerian (songino)   salad, already washed
-hulled almonds   flaked just enough.
Arrange the chosen smoked fish on the plate. Combine the valerian salad on top and season with evo oil and salt to taste. Finally sprinkle with a handful of peeled slivered almonds.

BAKED FISH WITH VEGETABLES

Ingredients:
-200g fish of your choice from fillets of cod, even frozen, or sea bream or sea bass
-100g cherry tomatoes (about 10)
-1 large zucchini
-Salt, parsley and oil
Arrange the chosen fish in a baking dish with baking paper, add the cherry tomatoes coarsely chopped earlier and then add the zucchini made into thin rounds. Drizzle everything with a drizzle of evo oil and then add the chopped parsley and salt and bake for about 20 minutes in a ventilated oven at 180 degrees.

EGGPLANT ZUCCHINI AND TUNA MEATBALLS

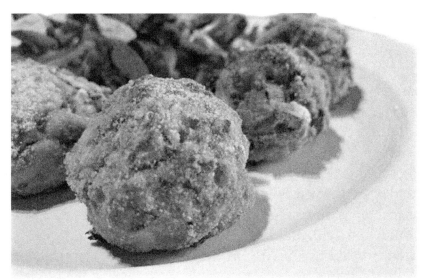

Ingredients:
- -1 small eggplant
- -1 small zucchini
- -2 cans of tuna without oil
- -1 whole egg
- -1 little bit of breadcrumbs

-Salt and parsley

Finely dice the eggplant and zucchini and cook them in a nonstick pan with a drizzle of evo oil and salt for about 10 minutes. Once cooked, drain the tuna and add it together with the finely chopped parsley and egg and mash them in the blender, make small patties with the mixture that has been created pass them on the breadcrumbs and place them in a baking pan with baking paper and finish cooking for about 15-20 min. in a ventilated oven preheated to 200 degrees.

BAKED COD MEATBALLS

Ingredients:
-150 g fresh or frozen codfish
-1 can of tuna without oil
-1 whole egg
-20gr of grated grana cheese
-parsley
-breadcrumbs oil and salt

Boil the cod by simmering it in a little water for a few minutes, then once cooked add the drained tuna, grana cheese, chopped parsley, egg and salt and puree in a blender. Afterwards take the mixture and form small patties, coat them in breadcrumbs and place them in a baking pan with baking paper and last bake until golden brown for about 15-20 min in a ventilated oven preheated to 200 degrees.

VEGETARIAN SPINACH AND RICOTTA CHEESE MEATBALLS

Ingredients:
-150g fresh sheep's milk ricotta cheese
-3 cubes of frozen spinach
-30g of grated grana cheese
-1 whole egg
-breadcrumbs oil and salt

Boil the spinach and then drain it and put it in a nonstick pan with evo oil and salt and sauté it for a few minutes.

Remove from the heat and let the spinach cool slightly, then put it in a bowl along with the ricotta, grana cheese and egg with a pinch of salt. Puree everything in the blender until it forms a smooth and soft dough, then form small patties, pass them over breadcrumbs and then place them in a baking pan with baking paper, last bake for about 20 min. in a ventilated oven preheated to 200 degrees until golden brown.

PROTEIN-FILLED ZUCCHINI (RECIPE WITH MEAT OR VEGETARIAN)

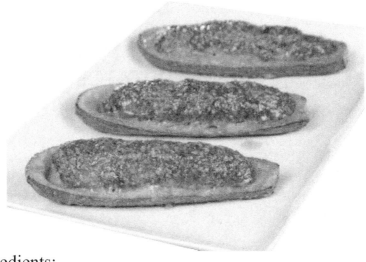

Ingredients:
-2 zucchini
-150g of lean mince or 100 g of feta for vegetarians
-6 cherry tomatoes
-30g of grated grana cheese
-1 whole egg
-Parsley oil and salt as needed

Wash the zucchini and hollow them out, extracting the pulp inside and then chop it into small pieces. Put it in a nonstick pan with the mince and the tomato previously made into coarse pieces and cook it. When the cooking is finished, add the grated parmesan cheese and the egg to the contents of the pan and puree in the blender and then fill the hollowed-out zucchini with the resulting mixture, then arrange it in a baking pan with baking paper and bake in a ventilated oven preheated to 250 degrees for about 20 minutes.

For the vegetarian version, hollow out the zucchini and sauté the flesh in a pan as above with the chopped tomatoes, remove from the heat and put in the blender adding the feta, grated parmesan cheese and egg, and blend until smooth. Finally stuff the previously hollowed out zucchini with this filling and bake as above.

GRILLED STEAK WITH POTATOES AND RED ONION

Ingredients:
-half a tablespoon of chopped oregano leaves
-half a clove of crushed garlic if liked
-30 ml white wine vinegar
-one tablespoon of olive oil
-200g rump steak, fat-free
-half a large potato cut into thick slices
-half a large red onion cut into thick slices
-about half a cup of arugula leaves
-1-2 lemon wedges before serving

The first thing to do is the marinating. To do this you will need to combine in a bowl by whisking with a fork: oregano, garlic, vinegar oil and salt to taste. Put the steak on a plate and pour the marinade on both sides of the meat. Let the meat cool in the refrigerator for 10 minutes and set aside the remaining marinade.

At this juncture blanch the sliced potato in boiling salted water for at least 5 minutes or at least until it begins to cook on the outside and is still firm on the inside.

Drain the potato and place in a bowl with the onion and remaining marinade. Cover them and set them aside.

Heat a nonstick skillet with a drizzle of oil over medium heat. Add the potatoes and onions while also combining the marinade and turning them until golden brown.

Continue to keep the pan hot and increase the flame to the highest setting. Now add the previously marinated meat and cook for about 6-7 minutes on each side until cooked to your liking. Remove from the heat and serve garnishing with the potatoes and golden onion.

 Later sprinkle the dish with the arugula leaves and add lemon wedges to taste.

SPICY SWORDFISH WITH AVOCADO SAUCE

Ingredients:
-half teaspoon of caraway seeds if liked
-half teaspoon of paprika
-1/3 teaspoon ground ginger to taste, less if desired
-a pinch of ground nutmeg
-a pinch of cinnamon powder
-half a tablespoon of oil

-1 swordfish steak
-rucola
-lemon wedges
Avocado sauce
      -half an avocado
      -1 tomato
      -1 sliced spring onion
      -a pinch of cilantro if liked
      -lemon zest and juice
      -half a tablespoon of oil

Mash the avocado with a fork and add the other ingredients for the salsa previously chopped up and pureed in the blender and refrigerate until needed.

Mix by whisking a little oil with the lemon juice and all the other spices with a fork and coat the fish with the mixture you have made.

Then heat the oil in a skillet over medium heat and add the fish and cook it for 2-3 minutes on each side to your liking.

Finally serve the dish with the avocado sauce and the addition of the arugula and lemon wedges.

ROAST CHICKEN WITH WINTER FRUITS

Ingredients:
-half teaspoon of chopped thyme leaves or your choice of 1 sprig of rosemary
enough olive oil
-one slice of chicken
-pitted prunes
-half a ripe pear
-half ripe red apple
-enough salt and pepper
-1 clove of garlic if liked

-1 teaspoon of honey
-half cup of white wine
-almond blossoms to taste

You can cook this meal the first time taking some time however you can play around with the quantities so that you can also save several portions to eat in the following days.

The first thing you need to do is to preheat the oven to 200 °C. Then combine the thyme leaves or rosemary with the oil and salt and pepper and garlic in one bowl.

Now take the shredded chicken and sprinkle it to season it in the oil with the herbs of your choice the salt and pepper and try to massage it in well to let it absorb.

Place the chicken in a nonstick baking dish previously covered with baking paper and then place in the ventilated oven previously preheated to 200 degrees and let it cook for one hour, turning it occasionally.

While the chicken is in the oven take the plums the apple and pear made into wedges and combine them with the white wine and honey in one bowl. Season and mix everything together making it blend as best as possible. Halfway through cooking, remove the chicken from the oven and arrange the fruit around the chicken, adding if you like 1 or 2 sprigs of thyme or rosemary and a drizzle of oil.

Finish cooking everything until the chicken is well cooked and golden, taking care to turn it as you go, and making sure that everything always remains fairly moist and adding a tiny bit of water if necessary.

When cooked, you can transfer the chicken and fruit to a platter. Let it rest for 15 minutes before serving.

All that's left is to serve the chicken with roasted fruit garnishing it to your liking with the almond slivers. You can also add a lemon wedge if you wish.

BREASAOLA BASKETS WITH CREAM CHEESE

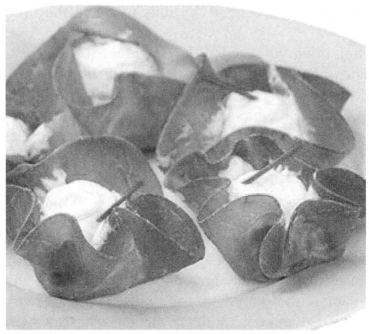

Ingredients:
-4   slices of bresaola
       -1 small block of light spreadable cheese also good in protein version
       -2 level tablespoons of grated parmesan cheese
-50   g arugula or lamb's lettuce, already washed
-a   tuft of fresh parsley
       -various seeds   for garnish with your choice of sesame or poppy seeds or flax seeds
-Plumcake   paper cups or metal kitchen ramekins

Put the spreadable cheese in a bowl along with the grana cheese and finely chopped parsley. Amalgamate afterwards and form 4 balls, place the bresaola on top of the ramekins and arrange the arugula inside and place the cheese balls in the center, then garnish with the chosen seeds and serve.

LIGHT VEGETARIAN PARMIGIANA

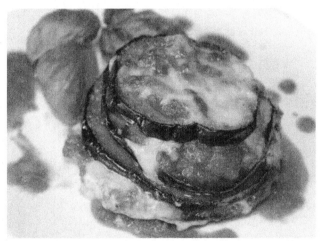

Ingredients:
-grilled eggplant or zucchini 200 g (you can also buy ready-made frozen ones)
-tomato pulp 200 gr
-1 mozzarella light
-30g of grated parmesan cheese
-1 tablespoon of evo oil
-enough salt
-fresh basil a clump
This very simple dish is an alternative to the classic parmigiana but in a light version.

You can decide to make it from either eggplant or alternatively grilled zucchini, and if you don't have time to grill them you can use ready-made frozen ones perfect for saving us time.

Shred mozzarella cheese and season tomato pulp with oil and salt to taste.

Take a small baking dish and arrange baking paper on it, then put a layer of grilled eggplant or zucchini, then on top with a spoon cover them with tomato pulp and a few basil leaves and scatter light mozzarella and parmesan cheese on top and then make another equal layer. Put a drizzle of oil on top and bake in a preheated ventilated oven at 200 degrees for about 20 minutes.

PROTEIN OMELETTE

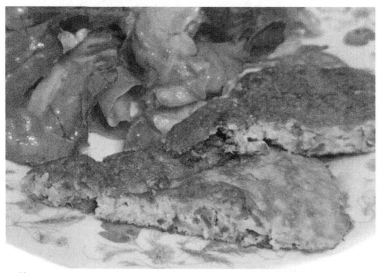

Ingredients:
-1 whole egg
-2/3 yolks

-8 chopped cherry tomatoes
-30g of grated grana cheese
-1 teaspoon of evo oil and salt to taste.

Combine the egg, egg white, grated parmesan cheese and salt and beat vigorously by hand with a fork. In the meantime pour the oil into the nonstick frying pan spreading it to the edges as well and add the previously chopped tomatoes over low heat for 5 minutes, then add the beaten egg and cover with a lid. After 5 minutes turn the frittata over and cook it well on the other side as well until golden brown.

To make a complete meal you can pair it with a nice salad with a slice of toasted whole-wheat rye bread.

You can also invent different fillings yourself by using, for example, grated parmesan cheese together with cubes of cooked ham or lean ham, or by adding pieces of chicken or filleted turkey, or in the vegetarian version by combining parmesan cheese, thinly sliced zucchini blanched in a pan or spinach or asparagus or lean cheese or other ingredients to your liking.

CHICKEN THIGHS IN SALMI' WITH OLIVES AND CAPERS

Ingredients:
- 4 skinless chicken thighs
- 40g pitted black olives
- 20g pickled capers
-1 clove of garlic if liked
- half cup of white wine
-2 level tablespoons of evo oil
- salt pepper and rosemary to taste

Take a nonstick pan put the oil and brown the garlic previously peeled, then put the chicken thighs rosemary salt and pepper and cook slowly fading with wine. If necessary also add a little water along with the wine cover with a lid and continue cooking turning the thighs from time to time. After about 20 minutes of cooking add the black olives and capers and finish cooking for another 15 minutes and serve accompanied by mixed salad.

SICILIAN-STYLE SWORDFISH

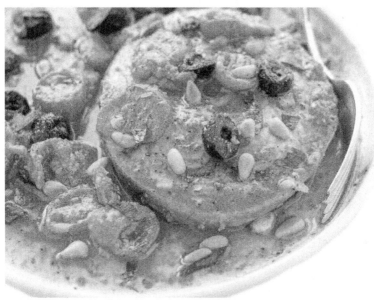

Ingredients:
- 2 slices of swordfish
- 10 pachino or date tomatoes
- 1 tablespoon capers
- 10 black or green olives
- a small cup of white wine
- origin as much as it takes

- enough salt
- Evo oil as much as needed
- caglio if you like

Take a nonstick pan and heat it after adding oil and if you like garlic. Add the cherry tomatoes previously cut into small pieces and brown them in the oil for a couple of minutes. Now add the swordfish slices placing them directly on the bottom of the pan and putting the cherry tomatoes around, now add all the other ingredients i.e. olives capers and oregano and salt to your liking.
Brown the swordfish 3 to 4 minutes per side and turn it over by deglazing with wine, cover with a lid, and cook for about 5 minutes.
Serve garnishing the fish with the cherry tomatoes and olives and the cooking capers and a sprinkling of oregano.

LEMON CHICKEN NUGGETS

Ingredients:
- 200g chicken breast morsels (take two slices a little high and shred into small pieces)
- 40g flour
- lemon juice and zest
- Evo oil as much as needed
- enough salt
- fresh parsley as much as needed
Take the chicken meat previously cut into chunks and mash them in a small bowl where you previously put flour and flour them, then take a nonstick pan where you previously added oil and onion if you like.

Add lemon zest lemon juice and a little water and add the floured chicken bites and a little salt and cook for about 10 minutes until golden brown.

When cooked, add fresh parsley and serve with a side of mixed salad.

LEMON SEITAN BITES

Ingredients:
- seitan 200g
- breadcrumbs as much as needed
- 1 lemon
- rosemary as much as needed
- 1 tablespoon of evo oil
- enough salt and pepper
- Sesame seeds as much as needed

Cut the seitan into thin strips, grate the lemon zest and grate it, then in a bowl put the lemon juice, oil, salt, pepper and sesame seeds. Soak the seitan in this mixture for a few minutes then coat it in breadcrumbs and brown it in the nonstick skillet until crispy. This dish can be served with a sprinkling of sesame seeds to taste.

CHICKEN OR TURKEY ROLL STUFFED WITH HAM AND CHEESE

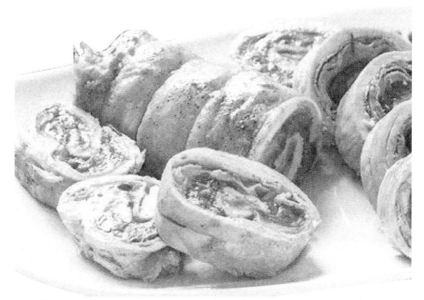

Ingredients:
- 300g thin slices of chicken or turkey breast
- 100g sliced cooked ham
- 100g of thin cheese such as scamorza or provolone
- a small cup of white wine
- enough salt and pepper
- rosemary and sage to taste
- Evo oil as much as needed
- kitchen twine

Take a piece of baking paper and lay the thin slices of chicken or turkey on it, side by side, overlapping them slightly, arrange the slices of cooked ham on top, trying to cover the entire surface of the meat slices, and again place the thin slices of provolone or scamorza cheese on top.

Roll all the ingredients onto themselves starting with one edge of the slices, also helping yourself with the baking paper until you form a tight roll that you will then tie with kitchen twine.

Place the roll on a nonstick baking sheet previously greased with evo oil and add rosemary and sage, salt and pepper to taste as seasoning.

Bake in a ventilated oven previously heated to 200 degrees for about 30 minutes until golden brown and remove from oven, serving to taste with grilled vegetables or mixed salad.

PROTEIN PANCAKES

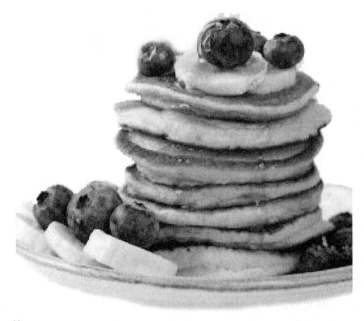

Ingredients:
- 100g low-fat Greek yogurt or natural white low-fat yogurt

- 55g flour
-100g of egg whites
-1 tablespoon brown sugar
-half teaspoon of baking soda
-lime few drops

Once the pancakes are ready, they can be stored for two or three days; in fact, all you need to do is seal them in a baggie, the kind used for freezing. You can then freeze and thaw them as needed. In this recipe, the dose is a bit more so that you can prepare them and then find them ready without having to redo them all the time, although the process is very simple and takes little time.

To garnish them you can indulge by using your choice of light fruit jam or otherwise jam with no added sugar, or protein hazelnut cream or some fresh fruit such as banana, blueberries, strawberries or raspberries with a drizzle of honey on top.

Place the egg whites in a glass bowl and beat them stiff with an electric whisk.

Then add the low-fat yogurt, flour, sugar and baking soda to the beaten egg whites and immediately add the lemon drops.

The baking soda reacting with the lemon will form a foam, at which point mix everything together so that the ingredients are blended until a thick and fluid batter is obtained. Then heat a not very large nonstick pan in which you can pour a drizzle of evo oil or a drizzle of coconut oil with the help of a kitchen brush. Then pour a ladleful of batter in the center and cook it for a minute and then turn it once golden brown, continue in this way for all the remaining batter by stacking the already cooked pancakes on top of each other on a plate.

At this point the pancakes are ready to be served topped to your liking, I usually choose one of the toppings I recommended above.

I also want to point you here to pancakes made with flavored protein oatmeal because I often make them myself and they are very good, I usually buy to make them the cookie flavored oatmeal or the ones flavored with apple pie or banana split or chocolate and cream cookie or there are many others and you can indulge yourself according to your personal taste.

Ingredients:

-100g egg whites

-30g of flavored oatmeal

-30g low-fat Greek or low-fat white yogurt

Beat the egg whites stiff with a whisk, then add once whipped the yogurt and slowly cascade in the oatmeal and continue to mix.

Once all the mixture is blended cook them in the nonstick pan as indicated above and garnish them to your liking.

LIGHT PROTEIN TIRAMISU

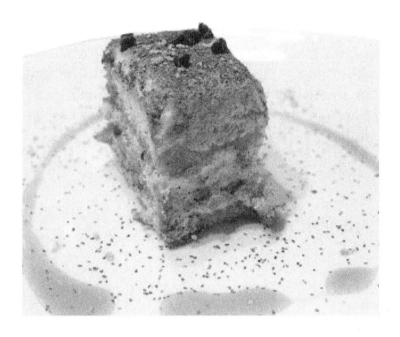

Ingredients for two servings:
- 2 single-portion packets of Pavesini cookies
- 1 cup of coffee
- 2 whole eggs
- 150g low-fat white Greek yogurt or 150 g light fresh cottage cheese
-2 level tablespoons of sugar
- stevia as much as it takes
- a pinch of salt
- bitter cocoa just   enough

Beat egg whites until stiff with a whisk, adding a pinch of salt, and refrigerate to chill. Prepare the yolk cream by beating the yolks with the sugar with an electric whisk until it forms a cream. Then incorporate the yogurt or cottage cheese into the yolk cream, mixing slowly. Slowly add the beaten egg whites and stevia to sweeten if necessary, lightly soak the Pavesini in coffee and then place in small bowls a layer of Pavesini and one of the formed creamy mixture, then yet another layer of Pavesini and another layer of cream, dust everything with bitter cocoa, chill in the refrigerator and serve.

COCOA PROTEIN PARFAIT

Ingredients for two servings:
-1 ripe banana
-150g low-fat Greek yogurt
-2 teaspoons of honey or stevia
-30g of bitter cocoa
-80% cocoa dark chocolate
-1 cup of semi-skimmed milk or soy or rice milk
Cut the banana into pieces and put it in the blender along with the yogurt and honey or stevia for sweetening. Next add the bitter cocoa and stretch it with the milk, adjusting to make sure the mixture is not too runny. Once a creamy consistency is reached, place the mixture in small cups to chill in the freezer for at least an hour. Serve after garnishing with the dark chocolate chips.

PROTEIN CHEESECAKE

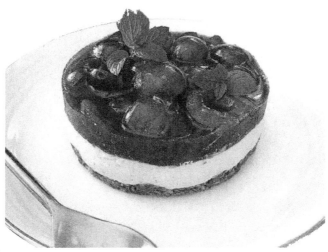

Ingredients:
- whole grain oatmeal 200g
- muesli 50g
- Milflower honey as much as needed
- fruit or natural low-fat Greek yogurt 250g
- light spreadable cheese 250g
- dark chocolate and chopped pistachios or almonds or hazelnuts to garnish

To prepare the base mix the whole grain oatmeal with the muesli in a bowl and crumble it, to do this mash it with the bottom of a glass and then add the honey that you have previously heated in a small saucepan over low heat making sure that the honey and cereal mix well.

Create a mixture and pour onto a round mold with a cheesecake opening, compacting it by helping yourself with a spoon.

Let stand in the freezer for half an hour.

Pour Greek yogurt and light cream cheese spread into a bowl and sweeten either with wildflower honey or stevia and mix well.

Take the mold with the cereal base out of the freezer and top it with the created cream, leveling it well on the surface.

Let the mixture sit in the freezer for a few hours to let it compact well.

When it is time to serve, decorate it with the dark chocolate previously melted in a bain-marie and the dried fruit granules of your choice and serve it cold.

Exercises to keep fit

Below are some simple exercises you can do at home to keep your body moving and healthy with the consequent activation of your metabolism, in fact doing physical activity increases energy expenditure, all of which will then go together with the beneficial effects of your new eating plan with an even greater improvement in lean mass at the expense of fat mass, to achieve even more easily the goal you set for yourself of getting fitter while staying healthy.

I offer simple exercises that you can do in sequence or separately to strengthen and tone all the muscles in your body.

You can repeat the sequences one or more times depending on your endurance or going then to increase them over time to intensify the workout.

Firming buttocks

I believe that having a high and firm butt is everyone's dream, and having a toned one is not impossible, in fact, you just need to do the right exercises to firm the buttocks, let's find out some of them together.

Rear gluteal slumps

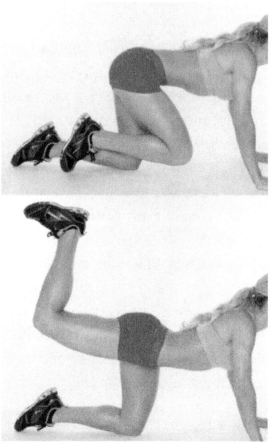

You can do this exercise either free-body or you may also choose to do it with weighted ankle straps or elastic bands, clearly increasing the effort and energy expenditure. Get on all fours and sprawl one bent leg backward with your hammer foot while maintaining a straight line with your back: then raise your leg past the line of your back and bring it back to the starting position. Repeat the exercise in sets of 15 2 times per leg.

Lateral gluteal slumps

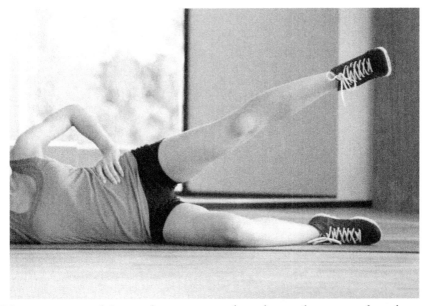

Lie on your side and rest your head on the arm that is on the ground. Bring your other arm to your side then raise your leg up and lower it without letting it touch the leg that is on the ground. Do 10 sets then switch sides and alternate leg and repeat for 3 sets.

Gluteal pelvis lift

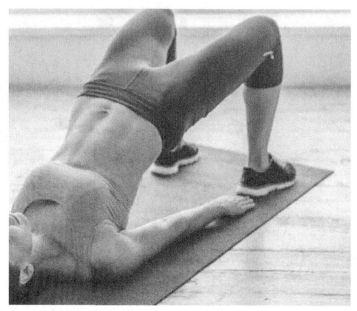

Stand on the floor with your arms along your body and bend your legs, leaving the soles of your feet in contact with the floor. Then raise your pelvis upward so that your body has a triangular shape and leave your shoulders attached to the floor. Lower your pelvis without letting your butt touch the floor and then raise again. Do repetitions of 15 for 3 times.

Inner Thigh Exercises

This is a specific workout for the inner thigh, to make it even more effective I use weighted ankle straps, but if you don't have them at home you can easily perform it without them.

The inner thigh is a trouble spot for some of us, but fear not, these are all simple and very functional exercises.

Exercise from lying down inner thigh

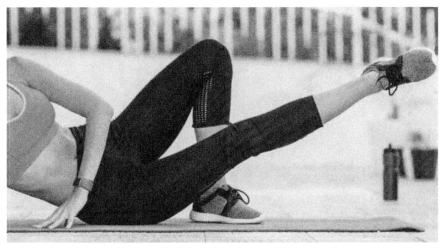

Lie on the floor on a mat and lie on your right side, with your right elbow resting on the floor and your hand supporting your head. Bend your left leg and place your foot and ground behind your right knee. Lift the outstretched right leg up and down while keeping the toe of the foot hammered down and then alternate the exercise on the other side.

Do the exercise for 15 lunges and repeat 2 times per side.

Legs up open and close for inner thighs

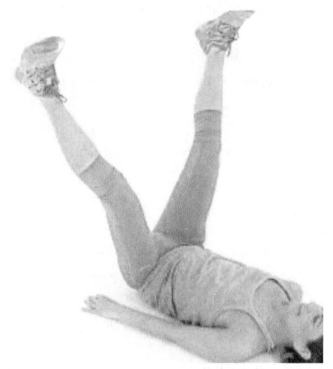

Let's continue firming the inner thigh with this other exercise.

Lie on the floor with your arms along your sides and bring your legs together stretched upward. Open and close your legs while keeping them extended. If you can, stand near a wall and move a few inches away from the wall with your pelvis and legs. Repeat 10 times the lunges for 2 sets.

Arm workout

Here are some exercises for the arms, which are in fact like the abs and buttocks a part of the body that we all dream of having toned, in fact unfortunately it is often the first to suffer the consequences of weight gain or low physical activity, it also suffers a significant loss of tone as we age.

Arm workout with chair

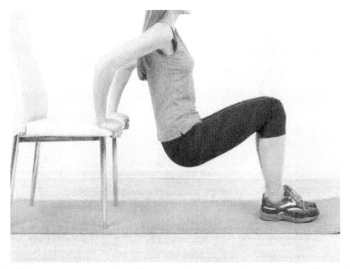

This dedicated upper body workout makes use of a chair.
In fact, to tone the arms, we do not always need large weights or special equipment; our own body weight is more than enough.

Rest your palms on the edge of the chair and put your legs in front of you with your feet resting well on the floor. Bend your arms and go with your pelvis toward the floor as far as you can taking care not to arch your back, which should remain as straight as possible. Repeat the exercise for 10 squats for 2 sets.

Arm workout with small weights

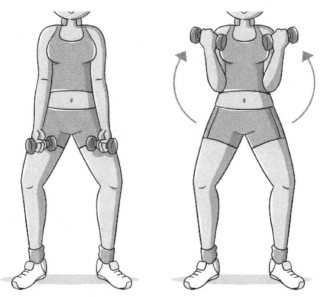

Here is another very simple arm-firming exercise that can be performed with small weights that you can find at Decathlon or many other sports stores, or even simple full water bottles are fine.

Start by standing with legs spread at pelvic height and knees slightly flexed.

Grasp the weights or water bottles with a firm grip and keep your arms extended. From this position, bend them toward your chest while keeping your elbows steady and then stretch them downward again.

As you perform the entire exercise strive to keep your back straight and your abs contracted to protect your lower back. Breathe in and out regularly and do not hold your breath, and perform the movements slowly. Do 3 sets of 10 repetitions.

Abs workout

The abdominals are a weak point for almost all of us as we often end up with an unsightly tummy, solving this problem may seem difficult but it is not impossible, so I propose ab exercises aimed at getting a flatter and toned abdomen that will improve even more by following the food plan recommended here, so much so that it will become a real healthier and more effective lifestyle to achieve the desired results.

Lateral abs

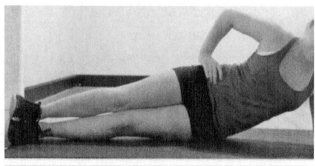

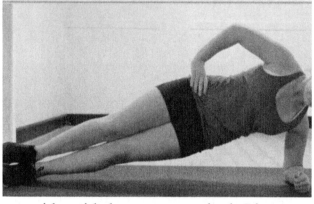

Lie on your side with legs outstretched. Place your elbow on the floor and your open hand on the floor. Lift yourself up by levering your side abdominal muscles and bringing your body up all at once. Now stay in this position keeping the muscles contracted for one minute and then come back down. Repeat remaining in the contracted position 3 times.

Bicycle floor workout

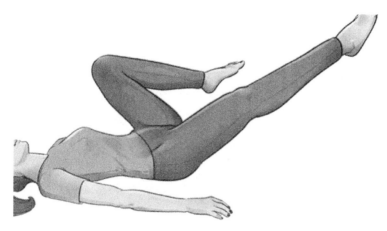

Lie down with your back on the ground and lift your legs up to simulate when you are pedaling a bicycle. Keep your arms along your sides and try never to touch the ground with your heels. This will contract your abdominal muscles, which will begin to work. Do the exercise for a few minutes.

Pillow abdominal workout

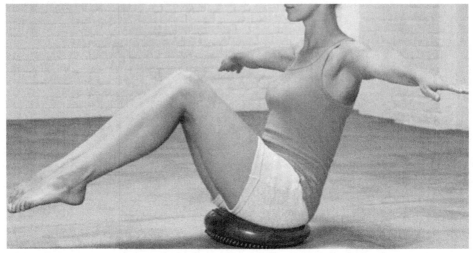

To develop balance and endurance, yielding tools are useful, even a simple pillow we have at home can be fine, alternatively you can buy soft rubber unstable bases like the one you see in the photo, which help us counteract body imbalance and maintain correct posture.

The work is on balance, so the abs are strengthened, but this exercise also comprehensively involves the entire body musculature.

Sit on the pillow and take your legs and feet off the floor and balance, stand still with your arms outstretched by pulling your abdominal muscles and holding the position as long as you can.

There are many ways to activate your metabolism, a very good way is to do it by keeping yourself moving with the right exercises like the ones I have given you some examples of above, you can then over time increase the number of sets to make your metabolism burn more and more. You can also vary the type of workout you do, such as going for a run sometimes or using the exercise bike or treadmill or going for a brisk walk outdoors, to make your metabolism be forced to adapt to different physical training situations. You can still change the times at which you exercise to prevent your body from getting used to the same rhythms all the time. All this is to create a strong synergy between the new eating plan you will adopt by following the Low Carb diet and physical movement, which will make achieving your goal of getting back in shape fast, soon a quick reality.

CONCLUSIONS

We have come to the conclusion of this journey. This book will be your little treasure, your secret weapon that you can use whenever you feel the need. Reread these pages every day and start cooking the various dishes I have described, begin this new journey that will allow your palate to enjoy and your physique to get back in shape.

If you want to have results, if you want to lose weight in a short time, you necessarily have to start taking action.

Probably everything you are doing or have done up to this point was not enough, if it led you to be dissatisfied with yourself. Probably if you have reached this point in your life you have been acting wrong for a long time, you have not taken the right path, for these reasons it is time to take charge of your life and give it a very strong steering. This book extends a hand to you to begin that food journey that will change you forever however it is up to you to try to hold on to that hand or not. If you don't, you will let yourself fall to the ground and you will hardly get back up.

It's time to change your eating habits and your way of thinking. You have believed for too long that you are destined to live in a body you don't like, instead you can change it as you see fit, what you need to do though is to feed yourself the right way.

For these very reasons you must immediately change your habits and replace them with positive ones.

As mentioned in the introductory chapter, everything I explained to you in this book I have applied day by day in my life. Before this type of diet I had tried others with poor results but this one for me was a real enlightenment. For these reasons I believe and hope that it can be the same for you, that it can finally help you achieve the fitness you have always wanted.

People in most cases hate diets because they believe they are very frustrating and that it is a process of continuous deprivation. Actually, if you learn to eat healthily and apply what I have told you, you will never feel the need to upset your eating plan. Your cheat days will serve you to get rid of the desire for some food that is bad for you, on the remaining days you will be able to eat healthy but also very tasty dishes.

Healthy eating does not mean living a life of deprivation or even less eating food without taste. Banish these thoughts from your head. There are chefs who have made healthy cooking their strong point. You have no excuse; you cannot even tell yourself that you do not have time to go on such a diet. In fact, there are plenty of dishes that can be prepared in a jiffy.

So identify your limiting thought that has so far prevented you from following a diet regimen or that has brought you back to even worse results than your initial state and break it down. Your strength lies in your mind before your body. They can present you even with a diet that worked for 99 out of 100 men, if you're not mentally ready, if you don't truly believe in what you're doing, you'll probably fall into the 1 percent of people who fail to achieve results.

This is definitely not the case with you because you went all the way through this book. You wanted to go deep into this topic and you did not let any detail slip through your fingers, this makes you different from most people. You should know that only 30% of people who buy a book make it to the end of it, if you have made it this far congratulate yourself, you are already different from most people.

The only advice I can give you at this time is to start immediately, if you have not done so yet, to eliminate all those bad habits and people who negatively affect your life, who become obstacles for you to achieve your goals. If every time you see someone in your family eating a very good but at the same time very caloric meal, you are sick, try to distance yourself or eat at a different time. You must never lose your compass, if you are mentally ready you can face this path with a smile, no one will be able to stand in your way.

Now is the time to choose what you really want to be in your life. Do you want to be content with your body that causes you to be dissatisfied, or do you want to live in a leaner body that is also more aesthetically pleasing to you? The choice is in your hands; I advise you to take the right direction and proceed without any fear.

The teachings in this book can prove to be very important in your life, don't lock them away in a drawer, you will only and exclusively harm yourself if you act that way.

In the first chapter I told you how important it is to love yourself before embarking on any path. Whenever you comment negatively about your physique, feel ugly, feel ashamed to go out and be in public, re-read that chapter, I really mean it. Finally begin to appreciate every aspect of you. Remember that no one is perfect but imperfections are precisely what sets us apart from others, instead of hiding them, enhance them.

Start daring, act differently, push yourself beyond any fear. It's time to get out of your comfort zone, change those bad habits that are ruining you day by day, overcome that wall that prevents you from living the way you really want. If you act differently, nothing worse can ever happen, and in case something doesn't go the way you hoped, you will have learned something new, you will have tried, you will have lived differently. Don't beat yourself up on the couch or your bed and counter your fears and problems with food, that is not the solution. Face life's issues head on, you have the broad shoulders to overcome them all. If you love yourself there is no point in doing things to please others. When you start a diet, you should not do it to reach the weight that others would like to see you at but to reach what you really want. You will then also become less inclined to do actions for the satisfaction of others, the pleasure to be satisfied must be yours first and then if others are okay with it you will be pleased, but if others think differently and judge you negatively for who you are this will not bother you. When you worry less about what others think you will have the freedom to really be yourself.

You will also begin to abandon self-pity once and for all; you will be aware that there will be days when you feel happier and others less so. You will know that your state of mind, your happiness and your well-being all depend on you. Happy people have the strength to find light even in dark days, in difficult times, they always manage to find an opportunity where others see only darkness.

You will not need to rely on others, because you will have the strength to rely on yourself, you will not feel the need to depend on other people. You will learn to trust your own abilities, yourself, you will know that you don't need anyone else to be happy, you won't need to show others how much you have changed or how much hard work you had to do to change, you will only improve to be at peace with yourself, and this will perhaps be your greatest satisfaction.

When you love yourself, you are able to make healthier choices that not only put you first but improve the quality of your life. It's time to be a little more selfish, to take time away from others or stop wasting it unnecessarily and devote it to productive activities for yourself. You can start resting properly, start exercising, start eating healthily, you are the sole architect of your success both physically and mentally. When you act this way you feel better, and the more you perform these actions, the better and better you will feel. You have no limits; you are the sole creator of your own happiness.

If you truly love yourself, you will not hold a grudge against your own wrong actions done in the past or even against those of others. You will have the power and all the cards to not only forgive yourself but also all others who have harmed you. You will be mature enough to accept any responsibility arising from your actions and to take any responsibility.

You will have all the makings of loving yourself and taking charge of your life. You will become more responsible for your actions when you learn to give more importance to your choices as well. You are the one who chooses how to live your life both good and bad. You are the one who decides what to eat and what not to eat; you are the one who decides what dietary regimen to adopt. You cannot complain if you are in a bad physical or mental situation; you only wanted it. It's time to make choices that are in line with your values, that allow you to honor them, that make you feel good, that don't really make you regret anything.

If you really want to live fully, I can assure you that loving yourself also allows you to emotionally bond in the best way with everyone else. When you live your emotions fully, when you dig deep within yourself, when you really understand who you are, there will be no one who can influence you. When you can open up and connect deep inside with others, without fear of showing your hidden parts, without fear of revealing your weaknesses, you will see everything with different eyes.

The moment you can raise your head, any fear disappears. Whatever is blocking you right now and preventing you from losing weight and getting into shape is only in your mind. Take an example from any person who has managed to lose weight and change his or her eating style throughout his or her life. Here you have my example in front of you, however there are many people in the world who have achieved great things. We all started from a difficult situation, yet at some point in our lives we have been able to fight back.

If you think I am telling you that all this is easy, my answer is, "no." If, on the other hand, you were to ask me if all this is doable, my answer would be, "yes." Now do you really want to let something within your grasp that could change your life slip through your fingers? I don't think so.

What I recommend, then, is to take the diet plan I have already given you in this book, select the meals you prefer from the different options I have given you for each day of the week, and start immediately. If you have bought this book you have set yourself a very important goal probably, that of losing weight and getting back into shape and firming your physique. You must never give up until you reach your ultimate goal.

Now that you have all the knowledge at hand all you have to do is act, you don't even have to think or procrastinate. If you keep procrastinating your actions and the start of your diet you are self-sabotaging, if you act this way don't complain if you find it difficult to achieve any result. Remember that only by taking action can you achieve a result. Only when you start giving importance to every food you ingest can you see results. As long as you stand still, you will not be able to achieve anything.

Now you are probably a different person than the one who started reading this book. You may have already read other books on this topic, but I hope this one can actually make a difference in your life. That is my goal, to stir people's consciousness with my personal story and to spread a teaching. Eating healthy and preparing tasty dishes at the same time can be done and most importantly, you don't have to be a chef.

I hope you will become a stronger, more ambitious person who loves herself with all her strength. Day by day with all the meals given in this book you will begin to see the first changes. Keep going until you achieve the fitness you dreamed of.

It's time to start your adventure...and remember that behind every success story is a person who made a courageous decision!

Best of luck!

AUTHOR INFORMATION

Claudia Rodriguez is a practitioner in the holistic field, specializing in self-help and nutrition, and works as a coach with nutrition counseling and support to help people regain their figure, health, and well-being.

Printed in Great Britain
by Amazon

26422535R00056